Married to a Stranger

An Alternative Approach to Simply Coping with Alzheimer's Disease

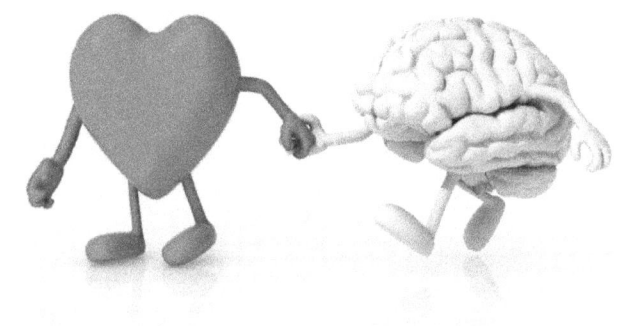

By Phyllis Lozeau

First published in April, 2016

ISBN-13: 978-1519692894

ISBN-10: 1519692897

LCCN:

Printed in the USA

Contents

Dedication

This book is dedicated to my six children and the millions of families coping with Alzheimer's Disease.

Poem about Alzheimer's
by Owen Darnell

Do not ask me to remember don't try to make me understand.

Let me rest and know you're with me.

Kiss my cheek and hold my hand. I am confused beyond your concept.

I am sad and sick and lost.

All I know is that I need you to be with me at all cost.

Do not lose your patience with me. Do not scold curse or cry.

I can't help the way I'm acting, can't be different though I try.

Just remember that I need you.

That the best of me is gone.

Please don't fail to stand beside me.

Love me till my life is done.

Author's Preface

Suddenly I found myself married to a stranger. This book is my testimony about what I have done to reverse some of the effects of Alzheimer's Disease for my husband of 60 years. It is our story. This should not be taken as medical advice.

Are you aware that there have been 21 drugs tested in nine years that have failed? This was reported in an AARP publication.

I have written this book because I believe that it can help others. Are you caring for someone with Alzheimer's Disease? Perhaps a family member is affected and you fear this may be in your future.

If you believe as I do, that God has given us everything we need to heal ourselves, then this book is for you and your loved one.

Part I

Is it Age or Something Else?

Chapter 1
Recognizing Alzheimer's Disease

Alzheimer's disease is like a thief in the night. It quietly creeps up on you and takes you by surprise. As we age, we can expect that we will not be as sharp. Occasional lapses in memory are universally accepted. Where did I leave my keys? What is that person's name? I forgot that I promised to call my sister! These examples all seem to be common as we age.

We no longer have to keep track of our days with a work schedule. We do not live by a time clock.

Sometimes the days run into one another so we don't remember what day it is unless we look at a calendar or our cell phone.

This is most likely just a sign of having too much going on. Or it could be caused by distractions or any of the four common reasons, which I will go into later. However, personality changes and things like forgetting to take medications or pay bills as well as obvious aggressive agitation can have serious consequences. When this occurs, it's time to get help and take action.

This book is meant for information only. Although I am a retired registered nurse, this is simply my documentation of my actual experiences in dealing with my husband's Alzheimer's disease.

I have always believed that God has already put everything we need to heal ourselves on this earth. We just need to find it.

This material is not intended to take the place of your doctor. The information should not be construed as medical advice. I can only tell you what I did and how it has affected my husband with full cooperation from his neurologist. Since we do not understand what causes Alzheimer's disease or what cures it, I began researching myself. According to a recent article in the AARP magazine, there have been 21 drugs tested in trials in the past nine years and all have failed to help an Alzheimer's patient. I went on a fact-finding mission - and yes, I prayed continuously to be led to the answers many sleepless nights.

The human body reacts differently, especially in the elderly, because we have had a lifetime to develop multiple diseases and wear and tear from our occupations and the environment.

Readers should always consult with appropriate health professionals on any health issue. Keep in mind that the medical profession is just beginning to recognize the benefits of herbal preparations. Doctors are trained to treat symptoms, not find the cause or the cure for diseases.

The pharmaceutical companies have made it their business to promote their own interest. Many incentives are given for prescribing their latest drug. When I see an advertisement on television and the side effects are plainly listed, it makes me wonder who in their right mind would want to take this. The food industry is just as guilty for their role in adding all the preservatives to increase shelf life, and also using artificial coloring and flavors to encourage sales. Both industries are profit driven.

Even our water is laced with fluorides. Civilization and population growth, as well as money motivation, has escalated all of these practices.

This has resulted in a huge boom with the organic food industry, herbal supplements and purified water.

Now research is proving that unsaturated fats and oils are a detriment to our brain health. The brain needs fat to function well.

What is happening in the brain of an Alzheimer patient? www.sciencedirect.com has some excellent articles on the genetic research being done.

Synaptic pathology is that which triggers memory loss. To understand the functions of the brain that are involved in memory and our thought process, it will suffice here to have an oversimplified overview.

The brain is very complex with trillions of nerve connections and billions of neurons (cells). Thought is transferred from neuron to neuron by an electrical impulse called a synapse. Each neuron has extensions called dendrites. The dendrites' function is to transmit and receive the electrical stimulus from the synapse.

In diseases such as Alzheimer's, the synapse are the earliest targets before building plaque and tangles. It is synaptic pathology that is the beginning of Alzheimer's disease and multiple neurological diseases. Once the scientists figure out how to prevent the synaptic pathology, Alzheimer's disease, Parkinson's, Autism, and Lou Gehrig's disease will be curable, or at least manageable.

The right frontal lobe mainly controls the memory, problem solving, impulse control, behavior, and emotions. The left frontal lobe controls speech and language.

The temporal lobes control the ability to recognize faces. The hippocampus is located under the temporal lobe. Long term memories, spatial navigation and emotional memories are stored in the hippocampus. When the hippocampus is damaged the patient cannot recall names, sometimes gets lost, and has difficulty with connecting emotional memories. This ability is critical to learning and remembering relationships. Alzheimer's disease causes the loss of remembering one's own children and eventually their loved ones.

Many toxins can penetrate the brain barrier as evidenced by neurological diseases. We recently received a report from our city water test that revealed that we have lead and copper in our tap water. Because my husband consumes a copious amount of water, I started to purchase purified water because of the fluoride. I am researching the type of filter to purchase to eliminate the lead and copper present in our tap water.

Chapter 2
Conditions that Alter Mental Status

Other ailments can also affect the brain function. We have to take all our diagnoses and potential diagnosis into consideration. As an example, diabetes can affect personality when glucose levels drop. One candy manufacturer has capitalized on the effects of dropping glucose levels by citing personality changes in their TV commercials. In reality this is not funny, but the commercial has humor and drives the point home. Incidentally there are over fifty conditions that can cause dementia.

Low oxygen levels associated with chronic obstructive pulmonary disease (C.O.P.D.) and severe sleep apnea are detrimental to the brain and the heart.

Poor circulation to the brain due to carotid blockages frequently cause changes in mental status.

Metabolic disturbances due to nutritional deficits are common because the elderly frequently do not eat well - especially when living alone or chewing with neglected dentures. These are a few that come to my mind that are quite common.

Many times we misinterpret confusion with the person having an undiagnosed hearing disability. The reader should be made aware that there can be other reasons that your loved one may exhibit similar symptoms to Alzheimer's disease. These symptoms should be investigated by a medical professional. Now research has shown that something as simple as a deficiency of vitamin D can cause depression and dementia.

In my years of nursing experience, I have seen a few misdiagnoses. Medicine is not an exact science. We all have wonderfully created bodies, but they do not always respond to treatment in the same way. It is important to communicate concerns with your primary care physician. Be sure the list of medications are in the medical history for the patient as well as any over-the-counter drugs. Include all herbal products as well. I wanted to rule out all the most common causes for my husband's symptoms. You could say that denial is a frequent response to a doctor when we do not want to hear the diagnosis of Alzheimer's disease.

Was my husband's medical history masking a more serious illness? My husband has been a diet controlled diabetic for years by using sugar free foods. Aspartame in sugar free foods has been known to damage memory.

He also has a severe hearing loss from working around heavy equipment that was used in our business for 30 years. Hearing aids do not always work, especially when one forgets to put new batteries in them. Answering a question inappropriately can be mistaken for confusion.

The hearing aid technician shared with me that when an individual has had a severe hearing loss as long as my husband has had, the brain forgets language and has to relearn it.

Several years ago he was diagnosed with sleep apnea, especially when sleeping on his back, which interferes with oxygen to the brain. It is detrimental to a healthy heart and brain.

It was discovered by his primary care physician in a routine physical that his heart rate was 38. This certainly caused lack of oxygen to his brain. At this time, he was experiencing mild angina and took occasional nitroglycerine. His family history of both parents included coronary artery disease, so his primary physician referred him to a cardiologist. The cardiologist did a cardiac catheterization and referred him to a heart surgeon after finding four blockages.

The cardiologist asked if Robert had early dementia when he discussed the results of the catheterization with me. My response was, "if you spoke to him through a mask, he never heard anything you said." Eventually it became obvious that this was a correct observation.

Chapter 3
Alzheimer's Disease Shows up in Everyday Life Situations

The evidence is there but often missed. The catheterization was at 8:00 am. At 5:00 pm I ordered him a meal, which did not arrive until 8:00 pm. By then he wanted his shoes. He was getting agitated and I thought he was attempting to leave.

Later I realized that his feet were cold, but he was having a problem with expressing that. His oldest son tried to calm him and he became angry. All this time I was thinking that we needed to get glucose into him, so I gave him a piece of cake with the frosting. When his meal came at 8:00 pm it also raised his glucose. He was fine personality-wise, but had to apologize for his verbal abuse.

Now, in retrospect, I believe that this was Alzheimer's disease just starting to show up - or perhaps a combination of both Alzheimer's with a low glucose level issue as well.

Unfortunately the heart surgeon was not available that night to follow up on the consult order as he was still in surgery at midnight with an emergency heart case. There were no contingency orders if the surgeon could not see him at a reasonable time.

The closer we got to midnight, the more I was demanding that the nurse get in touch with the cardiologist who was not on call at this hour (naturally). On-call doctors will not take it upon themselves to discharge a patient that they do not know. I could not afford to take him home against medical advice (A.M.A.) and not have the insurance pay for the cardiac catheterization. Certainly, I explained to the on- duty nurse that the insurance wasn't going to pay for an extra day for the convenience of a doctor either.

In the meantime, my dogs had been in the house for over twelve hours. She explained the situation to the on-call M.D.

The cardiologist himself called in a discharge order just before midnight. We saw the surgeon the next day for the consultation. In the meantime, I was recovering from open heart surgery (which I had five months prior with the same surgeon). Now we are referred to as the bionic couple.

May 2012 the surgeon made a decision to do an aortic valve replacement (frequently referred to as A.V.R.) due to his age (he had turned 80 in March 2012) and moderate calcified state plus a quadruple by-pass. It is important that the reader follow his course of events, as your loved one may be going through something similar and may have already experienced these symptoms or may develop them in the future. You might be feeling guilty that you may not have recognized it. I am medically trained and experienced in caring for the elderly and I was looking for a simple explanation. I myself didn't want to accept an Alzheimer's disease diagnosis.

Chapter 4
Surgery Affects the Elderly Adversely

It is not uncommon for elderly patients to experience confusion and agitation after having a long surgery, such as open heart surgery, from anesthesia. They are also subjected to medications that they don't usually take, such as pain medications and antibiotics.

On the first night Fentanyl was administered for pain intravenously. This drug has 46 known side effects. Since four grafts had been harvested from his legs, he had incisions from his groin down to his ankle on both legs as well as his chest. Every time nurses turned him he was instructed to self-administer the Fentanyl by pushing the button. He had not complained of pain, but the nurses, with good intentions, had him use it.

He hadn't eaten since midnight previous and kept asking for something to eat. Routinely the intravenous glucose sustains the patient. Vomiting is also a concern right after surgery so he was not allowed to have anything to eat until breakfast. This did not improve his disposition. I could see he was becoming more and more agitated. We explained the reasons to him numerous times in between his dozing.

Once he had breakfast he settled down. This is typical for diabetics to have some personality changes when they are hungry. He was well controlled at home with regular eating times with little variation.

The following may have been a result of post anesthesia, but I believe it was compounded by his Alzheimer's disease. The first day he had family in to see him, but he did not sleep. This was unusual for him. Normally, he could fall asleep as soon as his head hit the pillow. By sundown he had become very unmanageable. He just wanted to go home.

He even tried to pull out his central line. The frequent inflation of his blood pressure cuff also became a huge issue. There was just no reasoning with him. Three people had to hold him down to put on four restraints and then the surgeon was called for a Haldol (antipsychotic drug) order at 01:00 am. They do earn their money! This went on for over an hour. The Fentanyl was discontinued and Haldol was administered. He had to be restrained to keep him from pulling out his tubes and to help keep him in bed.

The next morning when I came to see him he started to cry and told me he thought he had done a terrible thing calling his daughter, son, and the night nurse awful things. Nothing could calm him until he called them on the phone to apologize.

He brought this incident up several times after being discharged. He still couldn't believe that he had been restrained. His recent memory was obviously still intact. Finally, he asked me if I would ever do that to a patient. I told him that nurses are legally bound to protect a patient from self-harm and I admitted that I had done this when necessary to prevent a patient from harming themselves. He never brought this up again.

Alzheimer's disease has a way of fogging our brain sporadically and it keeps the observer off balance. One minute the patient is totally lucid and the next minute they can be off-the-wall in their behavior. In retrospect, I believe that he was not only suffering from lack of sleep, but the Alzheimer's disease as well.

The cardiologist came in and asked him to identify him and gave him the surgeon's name as a test. Bob answered "you're the other guy". He could not tell the cardiologist his name, but at least he was aware of who he wasn't. He did remember his date of birth when he was asked, as is the protocol for a hospital stay. From then on, his recovery was uneventful until the night nurse gave him a prune juice and ginger ale cocktail for constipation.

I won't go into detail here, but I did wonder if he was confused - or just embarrassed? He could not find a plunger to fix things. Not a good thing for a post-heart patient to be trying to plunge a commode (definitely against doctor's orders). His method of cleaning up was a bit unconventional.

That is why we have housekeeping in the hospital. They are worth their weight in gold in a hospital setting. Most patients do get upset when they have accidents, but I never heard any of them tell the housekeeping staff "thank you". As a nurse I am eternally grateful for every housekeeper and Certified Nurse's Assistant that worked with me.

My husband quickly learned that the chair alarm would bring the nurses running when he stood up. I think he enjoyed all the attention he was getting. Even with this precaution, he did manage to get up and fall against the bed. Nurses earn their money too! He kept them running.

He never tried to pull on his chest tubes or other tubes again. He became the nurse's "dream patient" when using the walker in the hall. They had a hard time keeping up with him.

Anyone who has had open heart surgery knows the thickness of the instructions that one gets to take home.

On the sixth day, post-surgery, Bob was out riding his bike with the dog running beside him. He took the car and drove to Wal-Mart the next day - all against recovery instructions.

He did agree to drive the go-cart while shopping. I don't think the Alzheimer's disease was responsible for all of his noncompliance. He has always been a strong-willed individual. If you tell him he can't do something, he will figure out a way to do it anyway. Otherwise known as "bull headed" - or very resourceful.

It is safe to say that anyone with Alzheimer's disease does not listen to reason and will do pretty much what they want to do when they want to do it. This just compounded the issues as this was his nature to begin with. He is definitely a 'type A' personality.

Either patience is not in an Alzheimer patient's vocabulary or they simply forget what you just told them. There are times when this might be selective. Occasionally he chooses selective hearing. I know he has heard me because he jokes about it later.

I began to notice that he could never seem to remember the dog's name or that she was a female. She was a new family member to the family just prior to his surgery. He continued to call her by the male dog's name and tell her she was a "good boy."

Regardless of his noncompliance his recovery was the best that I have witnessed. His primary care doctor was amazed at how quickly he healed.

Perhaps there is something to be learned here. We might just be babying our post heart surgical patients.

Chapter 5
Searching for the Magic Memory Pill

I read everything that came up on my computer screen on holistic remedies that I was researching. I was interested in how many studies had been completed on everything I researched. I also wanted to know how many people took part in the studies.

Was there any independent testing done? Do they have a proprietary formula or the same amount of ingredients in every tablet? I decided to try Procera A.V.H.

Procera A.V.H. is a registered trademark for memory offered by The Brain Institute Research Lab. Procera A.V.H. is a proprietary, patented nutritional supplement. For more information go to www.ProceraHealth.com.

The dose is three capsules daily for memory and behavior improvement. I was surprised the order came with a book, which I have found to be a valuable resource. The book is, 20/20 BRAIN POWER by author Joshua Reynolds with Robert Heller M.D. Twelve experts with several letters after their names have written some very powerful comments on this book.

I use this as a reference. There are twenty seven pages of references in the back of this book with hundreds of chapters and pages listed to back up every claim made in the book.

On my second order I was gifted with a cookbook with beneficial recipes for brain health. I have used this as a guide for modifying my own recipes to include antioxidants for brain health.

Chapter 6
The Neurology Appointment

The neurology appointment was precipitated because of an aggressive outbreak in March of 2014.

The toilet had overflowed at midnight and my husband could not find what he was looking for in the garage to repair it. I was trying to convince him to just shut the water off and repair it in the morning. At that time two of our visiting children arrived home and tried to calm him with a promise that my son would fix it in the morning.

Our children were fearful that he was going to hit me because he was so aggressive and was verbally abusive. This was a complete personality change for him.

They went into another room until he calmed down and went to sleep. The next morning all was forgotten. He fixed the toilet like nothing ever happened. This agitation is so typical of early Alzheimer's disease. This is when I started the Procera A.V.H. It improved his mood within an hour and his old personality returned after the first dose.

He had been taking the Procera A.V.H. for a few weeks by the time we saw the neurologist and it had not improved his memory at all. The memory takes time to improve as new brain cells have to replace old damaged neurons, dendrites and synapse.

Having his normal personality back made it worth the cost, but he was not able to answer any of her questions. He did not know how many children he had, their names, his address or his birthday. He could not tell her the President's name or the season.

This was an obvious decline in his mental state since his surgery in May of 2012. She prescribed Namenda to prevent further progression of Alzheimer's disease and Aricept for memory. You may think, what could be worse?

Some patients forget how to dress themselves and how to feed themselves. They progress to incontinence and do not remember toileting at all.

Some sleep days and some are up all night. They just exist in a vegetated state. Fortunately, he could still care for himself.

Depending on what parts of the brain are affected controls the behavioral effects we see in the patient. Sadly some forget who their spouses are and pursue other romantic relationships when confined to a facility.

It is not uncommon to have episodes of paranoia with sudden mood swings. It is necessary to not take these personality changes personal when they are directed toward family members. Hurt feelings are easier to ignore when one realizes it is the disease causing these outbreaks. You will find yourself taking on the role of an ambassador and having to smooth ruffled feathers from time to time.

The disease eventually destroys the part of the brain that controls breathing and heartbeat until they pass away.

It doesn't matter how bright or talented one is - no one is immune to the effects of the disease. You may recognize a few names on the following list. These folks had the best care money could buy, but also suffered from Alzheimer's disease.

- Norman Rockwell, the painter famous for Saturday Evening Post magazine covers
- Mabel Albertson, actress in Bewitched
- Rita Hayworth, actress in the 40's
- Sugar Ray Robinson, professional boxer
- Aaron Copland, composer
- Burgess Meredith, actor who played Rocky's trainer

- Thomas Darsey, Gospel musician,
- Betty Robinson, Olympic medalist,
- Joe Adcook, professional baseball player,
- Perry Como, singer
- Charles Bronson, actor
- Ronald Reagan, actor & former President
- Carroll Campbell, Governor of S. Carolina,
- Charlton Heston, actor with multiple Oscars
- Peter Falk, actor from Columbo TV series
- Pauline Phillips Van Buren, author of Dear Abby Column
- Glen Campbell, country singer, composer with 5 Grammy Awards
- Malcolm Young, rhythm guitarist
- Jimmy Stewart 5 Academy Awards for best actor
- Estelle Getty, the actress who played Sophia on the Golden Girls

Looking at this list it is safe to conclude that it has nothing to do with intelligence or an inactive brain, as some have suggested.

Chapter 7
The Astronomical Price of Alzheimer's Disease

There are 5.4 million people who suffer from this debilitating disease. This affects their families as well. This disease ranks sixth in the cause of death. It is estimated that over 148 billion dollars are spent each year treating them - without any noticeable success.

At the rate that our aging population is growing, it is estimated by the year 2050 there will be almost 14 million people living with this condition.

Presently, there are no pharmaceutical cures on the horizon to actually halt or reverse the symptoms. So far the focus has been on destroying the plaque that forms and nothing on prevention that I am aware of.

Namenda may slow it down, but it does not hold much promise of halting or curing it. The cost of Namenda is $144 a month with part D insurance once you are in the "donut hole". The drug costs are just the "tip of the iceberg". The cost of confinement will put the family in the poor house. This is what has prompted me to take an alternative approach with the goal of avoiding confinement.

Aricept did not work for my husband - he had no improvement in his memory. Robert was on Aricept for over a year and could not hold a conversation. He had no word finding ability. It was very frustrating for me, as well as him, to figure out what he was trying to tell me.

I changed him to Bacopa in April 2015 (a Himalayan Herb). After he took it for 7 nights at bedtime, on the eighth morning, he began to tell me of all the experiences he had when my dad worked for us. This lasted 30 to 45 minutes. I was blown away. He never missed a word and he made perfect sense.

Bacopa has also been recommended by Dr. Oz. on his television show. It is also recommended in several of the books I've read on natural treatment. It improves mental clarity and has a tranquilizing effect, even though it enhances focus and memory. Bacopa is an antioxidant. It protects the brain from free radicals. Bacopa improves mental clarity and increases the efficiency of nerve impulse transmission. Bacopa supports attention, learning, memory, relaxation and calmness - as well as a positive mood and emotional well-being.

There are times that my husband will call things by the wrong name, but when I question him, he thinks about it and gets it right. He has improved 90% in his communication skills. He still has off days now and then.

Why am I so in favor of herbal supplements? I have not seen any evidence so far where a drug has worked satisfactorily, in my opinion.

Think about it for just a moment. Chemical fertilizers and pesticides rob the soil. Top that with the refineries that take most of the nutrients out during the processing of our food; we may as well be eating cardboard.

There is nothing left in white flour as compared to the whole grain content or the bread our grandmothers made. Industrialized civilization had not yet taken its toll on their generation.

Previous generations had no need for working out or taking yoga classes. Daily chores were necessary to survive. To top all that off, firewood warmed you twice. Once when you cut it and again when you burned it. Most people did not have automobiles, so they walked. The children were active and not couch potatoes with their video games - like in today's society.

My dad always had a garden and hunted, fished, and raised his own meat. We were raised on organic produce - not even realizing the benefits. Crops were rotated and fertilized the old fashioned way. No chemicals were used. There is a method of planting onions between the crops to prevent insects from ruining the vegetables. Jerry Baker has authored several books on gardening tricks using products we use every day. His newest book is on all the foods you find in the grocery store to heal everything that could possibly ail a human. You may have guessed by now that I love books that help to keep us healthy.

Chapter 8
Drug Trials

I have refused to put Robert into a drug trial study. As I stated before, we do not know the exact cause or the cure for this dreaded disease, but we are getting closer thanks to the companies who are researching potential natural cures.

I am doing my own study with natural products by keeping notes on the results. I believe there are several factors that contribute to Alzheimer's disease so we need to take multiple approaches.

I have added only one thing at a time, monitored the results and observed how it affects him.

After several months on Procera A.V.H. I wanted to know if it was doing him any good or if it was the Aricept and Namenda. I stopped giving him the Procera for seven days. This turned out to be a big mistake on my part.

He became agitated with the co-volunteers who we were working with at a charity for the needy through our church. I had to take him home. It was obvious that the procera had worked. I ordered it that afternoon.

A few days later my oldest daughter was coming from Vermont for her brother and sister's birthday.

I waited until six am to tell him that she was flying in that day.

By 8:30 he was ordering me to get in the car to get her even though her flight was not landing until 1:30 p.m. He was very aggressive and I could not reason with him. I tried to explain that it was only a half hour trip to the airport and we could not leave the dog in the car or take her into the airport and wait over four hours.

He missed two exits to the airport before I finally got him to turn around and head back home. He seemed to be a bit calmer as he started to recognize landmarks. By the time we arrived home it was time to make lunch. Miraculously, my Procera order came in the nick of time, and I gave him the daily dose after his meal.

After lunch we left for the airport and by the time she landed, he was his old self. This change in personality was noticed about an hour after taking the Procera. Needless to say, I will keep giving this to him. I can't chance having such a radical change in his personality. It could be a danger to me.

Procera A.V.H. - the A stands for acetylcarnitine, a neurotransmitter enhancer, which helps increase brain blood flow and circulation and supports mitochondrial function.

Vinpocetine is derived from the natural extracts of several plants, including the periwinkle flower. It helps support blood flow, raises oxygen levels and boosts cerebral metabolism; thus affecting the personality change. It is also an antioxidant which protects the brain against neurotoxins and stress as well as alcohol and poor diet.

Huperzine, also known as chinese moss, is a natural acetylcholinesterase inhibitor. Quite a mouthful for an enzyme that destroys acetylcholine in the synapse before it's effectively used to form your thoughts and feelings.

The focus of the drug study is on the amyloidal plaque that forms in the brain of the Alzheimer's patient. I don't know of any studies being done to rebuild; neurons, dendrites, synapses or improve memory. Studies are ongoing to discover the functions and how the synapse and neurons work.

There is evidence that antioxidants in organic foods are beneficial. I am addressing foods and recipes to nurture the brain in a future chapter entitled "Scrub Your Brain with Nature's Antioxidants".

The neurologist recommended B12 as a result of the low level in his blood. I added DMAE (Dimethylaminoethanol Bitartrate) 351 mg. for memory to enhance mental concentration. DMAE is a precursor of acetylcholine, which is a key neurotransmitter in the brain. This is not impossible to pronounce if you separate the syllables. 'Di-methyl- amino- ethano Bi- tar- trate'.

After 30 days I did not see any improvement, so I discontinued it. This may be effective for some, but not in his case.

Other herbal products he takes are Turmeric Supreme - one in a.m. and one at bedtime before sleep for his arthritis. This has replaced Aleve (which he took two caps twice daily).

It is believed that inflammation of the brain contributes to Alzheimer's disease.

Turmeric Supreme has many benefits. It's being used as a painkiller because of its anti-inflammatory properties. There are many studies on turmeric at this time. I recently read a report that turmeric enhances cognition by protecting the cells. It has the ability to bind with and dissolve abnormal proteins. It's nature's mood enhancer. Be sure to read the ingredients before you purchase any. One drawback was that turmeric was not being absorbed well by the body. Most products now have piperine, a black pepper extract, which facilitates absorption so that the turmeric gets to the cells where it can be utilized.

The Cancer Center gives turmeric to prevent nausea caused by chemotherapy.

Cod Liver Oil with vitamin A and vitamin D is one of the best sources of Omega 3.

It was first used medically in 1789 by Dr. Darby of Manchester England for rheumatism and in 1824 for rickets because of the Vitamin D content. It is believed to be beneficial in preventing atherosclerosis and lowers the progression of coronary artery disease.

It has been suggested that it may improve cognition in aging brains associated with the link to vitamin D. I have added D3 10,000 IU for his psoriasis and the benefits to his brain. I have also added B6 and folic acid with the B12

Just prior to publishing this book I have found Vectomega. One tablet is equal to six ounces of salmon and is 50 times more absorbable than fish oil. This is backed by clinical studies. I have not yet tested this on Robert to see the effects. For more information, visit www.Vectomega.com by EuroPharma. The literature states it is for a healthy heart, brain function, cellular health and healthy inflammation response. It's free of heavy metal contamination, cholesterol and toxicity.

Continually staying on top of research is key. I will seek information from other sources before adding Vectomega.

Robert's Medications:

Baby Aspirin 81 mg. prescribed by his cardiologist, for heart health as a blood thinner. Recently I have discontinued the Aspirin as the Cod Liver Oil thins his blood and he was bruising too easily. As stated above, I am considering changing to Vectomega as a source of Omega 3. I work with the physician's P.A. when changing anything and I update his records.

Namenda, 28mg. daily, has been prescribed by his neurologist to prevent the advance of Alzheimer's. It's the only medication for Alzheimer's disease that he is taking presently.

I want to recommend downloading the Alternative Daily Publication on coconut oil. There are multiple resources listed. This can be downloaded for a minimal fee online. Coconut oil has multiple health benefits, especially for the brain.

Dr. William Campbell Douglass II's book, "The Free Man's Declaration for Health and Longevity." He has spent over 40 years treating patients all over the world - sorting out "junk" medicine and he states, "I have seen firsthand how political red tape and corporate profits can interfere with medical discoveries. In my opinion, this is an egregious lack of integrity."

This book has become a valuable resource for my research. He covers multiple illnesses. I purchased his book online as well.

The Brain Research Lab sent a book with my first order of Procera A. V. H. - "20/20. Brain Power" by Joshua Reynolds with Robert Heller, M.D.

"Miracles from THE VAULT Anthology of Underground Cures" by Jenny Thompson of Health Services Institute. These publications have been my main source of information. They are written so the non-medically trained public can comprehend. The Health Service Institute has done research for eighteen years on herbal products. I have full confidence that they are experts in the field of natural remedies.

Dr. Mark Stengler's Natural Healing Encyclopedia is another excellent reference book. He is a family board certified physician. His clinic is in San Diego where he practices holistic health, alternative naturopathic remedies.

He is an expert in nutrition, herbal therapy, vitamin therapy, homeopathy, and natural hormone replacement. He recommends seven herbs for memory health. Phosphatidylserine, Bacopa, Ginkgo Biloba, B12, Huperzine, Flaxseed Oil, or Fish Oil, and Acetyl-L Carnitine. Amazingly I had found five out of seven of these through research on the internet before purchasing his book. I was encouraged by this confirmation that I was on track.I have spent hours researching many articles online. According to the University of California in Los Angeles, spending time online doing research is a form of brain exercise. Nice to know. I always search the credentials of the individuals and read all the testimonials from the consumers. I realize that we can't always believe everything that is on the internet because we don't know the writer's motives. It's my opinion consumers have the most credibility.

I have not tried jellyfish extract yet. You may call 888-565-5385 or look up Prevegan www.prevegan.com for more information on this newest discovery.

Part II
Progress Inch by Inch

Chapter 9
Improvements

I have made progress with Robert's behavior and communication skills. He has not forgotten how to fix everything around the house. He was a builder in the winter months for 30 years and a swimming pool contractor in the spring to fall season.

I have to admit that his workmanship has slipped some. He has forgotten that concrete sets up quickly in the July heat. He was skilled in finished carpentry, masonry and designing.

He still has trouble putting names and places together but knows where he has to go to get material to complete his projects.

I refer to this as "not connecting the dots." At times he loses focus when someone is conversing with him about a particular person - especially if the story is long. He does better with shorter conversations. He is able to joke and retain small sequences of events. When giving him directions, I find that only one thing at a time works best - especially when he is looking for something or asking him to put an item away.

I realize that rebuilding neurons, dendrites, and the synapses for thought processes takes time, so I am expecting more progress in the area of short term memory. I have not known of any motor skills being affected by Alzheimer's disease.

He always helps with the household chores. His reading comprehension has improved. Now he can read a magazine or newspaper and stay on task. I'm not sure how much he remembers of what he reads though. He has shown interest in the list of things he needs to remember.

He knows his children and their names in a photo and when they visit. Sometimes accurately, sometimes he mixes them up. When you have six children, you sometimes go through a litany of names before you get to the right name even without Alzheimer's disease. He still has trouble remembering which grandchild belongs to which child. He does know the ones who live in our vicinity that he sees more often.

I frequently have him look at the photos that the family puts on Facebook. Recently a photo of his mom and dad with his family and himself was on Facebook and he knew all of their names. He shows interest in Facebook postings of videos of children and animals as well as family photos. He watches for at least an hour at a time.

Patience is something we, as caretakers, have to develop. It is somewhat like having a four year old in an adult body. Repetition is a friend and has to be applied on a daily basis. I have noticed that he naps several times a day. He has a schedule similar to a baby. I am thinking that he is regenerating parts of his brain like a baby is growing. Perhaps, I am rationalizing but there is always a hopeful possibility.

We are going into our second year on the herbal routine and I see a tremendous improvement. It is my earnest wish that this book is helpful to other caretakers of Alzheimer's patients. We have to take it a day at a time and be very grateful for our little victories.

I regret that I did not start sooner - instead of trying to rule out other causes of his dementia. Keep your loved one involved with other people and events and functions as much as you can. Sometimes children can play simple games with them. It is a joy to watch the interaction with a pet or a child. They might even be encouraged to read a children's book to the child. It is therapy for them and the little ones love it.

Chapter 10
Be Grateful for
Every Little Victory

There will be days when there are setbacks. Do not despair. Learn to have joy in the small victories. The following is an example of how my husband reacted to a crisis.

Our youngest daughter had a near-death emergency. She had a ruptured aneurysm with a dissecting aorta. Her fiancée got her to the hospital where the family quickly gathered. Her dad held her hand and cried.

Amazingly, he knew the seriousness of her condition. While she was having a C.T. scan done in the E.R., my husband joined her fiancée and myself in prayer. She was not expected to survive by the medical staff, but by the grace of God, she did. Arrangements were made to have the air ambulance fly her to Orlando from Daytona.

I had to get to Orlando to take care of paperwork for her admission. He chose to stay with his daughter rather than return home until the helicopter crew took her for a twenty minute flight to Orlando.

This was most likely the most lucid moment that he had experienced in a year. Considering the stress level that we were all experiencing, the way he reacted was nothing short of a miracle for an Alzheimer's patient. She is one of the 2% to survive and did get to come home after nine days in intensive care.

Robert was trying to be a help by organizing her garage. We had to stop him because she wouldn't be able to find anything later. He still puts things where you least expect to find them.

This is common with an Alzheimer's patients.

This May he is giving her away. She has never been married. It will be a dual celebration for her survival and her wedding day. He is looking forward to wearing his tuxedo.

He has misplaced his wallet twice now. He has since found the second one - right where he placed it, in a bathroom draw. This was after replacing all his crucial information.

He does not drive without me. If his driving skills change, I will take over the chauffeuring. Now I keep his license in my purse and he has no debit card. I have taken over paying for everything. Make sure to keep copies of the Alzheimer patient's important cards that are in their wallet.

I never find my pots and pans in the right place, but he tries to put them where they belong. Living with an Alzheimer's patient is definitely a challenge. You have to expect to double check for faucets left running, burners left on, and toilets not flushed.

In his early stages, I came home and smelled something burning. The coffee pot was on the stove reheating and on fire. A few times I have found faucets still running and the refrigerator door not closed.

More than once we have spent time looking for his hearing aids, glasses or misplaced keys.

I had to find excuses for him not to put clothes in the wash after he put bleach instead of soap in a load of dark clothes. We have a wardrobe of tie dyed jeans now. It is useless to tell someone with Alzheimer's disease they did something wrong because they just do not remember and will tell you, "I never did that or I never said that."

I have gotten creative in finding little chores that he can accomplish to keep himself busy because he has been very active all his life. My husband loves to fix things. He hates puzzles, but will spend hours figuring where the pieces go from a broken vase.

He still rides his bike while the dog runs along with him. He attends church with me and understands the sermon - especially when the pastor makes a comical reference to his family life.

He is able to drive and knows where he is going. He may not know the name of the store or restaurant, but he knows what he wants to buy.

I do not let him go alone to get groceries anymore or I will end up with about $30.00 worth of foods that we don't eat.

When giving him money, I only give him ten dollars at a time. You will learn, or may already know, your loved one's habits. It gets easier to prevent disasters after a short time. He spent nearly 58 years taking care of me in many ways, so now it is my turn. We have been married 60 years as of September 2015.

Recently he knocked over a full cup of coffee, and then proceeded to wipe it up. After wiping up the spilled coffee, he tried rinsing the dirty rag in my clean dish water. This was way out of character for him. As a young man, he ran the pasteurization and clarification of milk in the family dairy. His job required sterility procedures which were second nature to him when he was well.

On two occasions he exhibited symptoms of paranoia. None of us were able to comprehend what triggered the paranoia. For some unknown reason, known only to himself, he was angry with his youngest son and refused to hug him when he was leaving. All he would say was "he knows what he did". In actuality, our son hadn't done anything to anger him.

The remarkable thing was that he told me about this on Friday and again on Sunday about people who had been visiting us earlier in the week. This was evidence of recent memory.

My son stayed away for a month. When he did come to visit recently, my husband met him at the door and apologized profusely, with tears welling up in his eyes. He told his son he did not know why he acted so crazy. Again, this negative incident was recent memory and ended with a hug and forgiveness. It was a very emotionally charged scene.

Another time my daughter's fiancé' came to fix my computer without my daughter. Apparently, Robert did not recognize him. When her fiancé Todd was leaving I gave him a hug. Bob appeared to be asleep so Todd did not say goodnight to him. I walked my future son-in-law to the door so I could lock the door and put out the lights. The next morning you would have thought I was having an affair with this man. Again, on the positive side, this is recent memory; however, distorted.

Later we all had a good laugh about this, including my husband. Unfortunately, this was a case of not recognizing a familiar face.

The next time he came I made sure he came with my daughter. Robert has been fine with him ever since.

Dr. Glen S. Rothfield, author of "The Atlas of Natural Cures" recommends blood tests to determine vitamin and hormonal deficiencies as well as the presence of heavy metals. All of these can contribute to Alzheimer's disease if not within the normal values.

Chapter 11
Scrub Your Brain with Nature's Antioxidants

God has given us everything we need to heal ourselves. Unfortunately, our fast pace of living has lured us into fast foods. These foods are prepared with chemical names we cannot even pronounce and loaded with preservatives for long shelf life. This amounts to big profits for the food industry.

We have even added junk foods and high sugar drinks in our schools. As a society we continue to punish our bodies with unhealthy habits.

On the positive side, wine is beneficial in moderation. There is an emergence of health food stores and companies interested in the longevity and health of their consumers. If you think organic foods are expensive, compare the cost to the confinement cost of an Alzheimer's disease patient.

The key is to eat fresh fruits and vegetables grown without pesticides and chemical fertilizers, meats grown without antibiotics and pure water not contaminated with chlorine, fluoride, metals or bacteria. I have invested in a filter to remove toxic metals and a solution to remove fluoride and chlorine.

After 21 days the desire for junk foods will be gone. Everyone who adopts better eating habits will feel better and may even lose a few excess pounds in the process. I have streamlined and tweaked my meal preparation to include several servings of greens like kale and arugula - plus our usual spinach, beet greens, and green beans every week.

I use red onions with sweet peppers and mushrooms in stews or on the side. Plan your meals with Alzheimer's disease in mind.

There is a diet available from the Memory Healer Program that you can order online. The diet gives a specific amount of each group of foods depending on the chemical makeup in combinations to be eaten at a specific time of day. The chemicals necessary for the brain are in the suggested foods.

I would attempt this diet, but my husband would never accept the rigid routine for 21 days. There is a tremendous amount of variety, but it requires discipline.

I do disagree with one opinion in this publication reference in regard to herbal products not being of any benefit. I disagree because of the fact that I have seen the tremendous improvement in my husband and an immediate decline when I changed his routine supplements.

Without going into detailed chemistry, I have created meals that disappear off the plate using multiple variations. I have spent many hours on the computer researching antioxidant rich foods.

I have recently added Lion's Mane capsules. There is research and several consumer testimonies of the benefits of Lion's Mane. This is a mushroom also available in tablet form. I have also added generous amounts of Kale, Spinach and Arugula to my recipes. Adjustments have been required to regulate my own blood thinner medication to be able to include these greens in my diet as well.

I added berries to deserts and cereal and even salad, baked foods, as well as flax seed. I cook with coconut oil and olive oil daily. I have substituted oatmeal that I grind in my coffee grinder and barley as an exchange for less white flour in pancakes and baked foods. Additional eggs are added for increased protein and ½ tsp baking soda in these recipes.

We eat as much organic fruit and vegetables as possible, and have added smoothies to our daily routine. If your mate or parent has high cholesterol, Wal-Mart has a great tasting Egg Maker that taste as good as eggs. Canned foods have just about been eliminated. I use the pressure cooker and the steamer for fresh vegetables.

Every day has been fun to see the new creations. Lucky for me, my husband is not a fussy eater. He did draw the line when I served him scrambled eggs with kale. Yuk! The green eggs were not appetizing. Sorry Dr. Seuss! Now I make omelets and put the vegetables inside.

Diabetics ingest aspartame for years in sugar free foods. Aspartame has been associated with loss of memory. We have switched to stevia, a natural product, as a sweetener.

Cinnamon has been shown to be a benefit in aiding sugar metabolism and has also been shown to improve memory. I put it in our oatmeal and on our toast with stevia.

I recently added bottled water to our grocery list to avoid the fluoride in the city water. I read labels on the tooth paste. All of this may seem like it's overboard to some of you, but when you live with an Alzheimer's patient you find yourself analyzing everything you eat and drink.

Years ago cooking with aluminum pans was suspect. Now we rarely see a pan made from aluminum.

Chapter 12
Recipes that I Have Modified for A.D.

Vegetable Lasagna

Adjust amounts if you are cooking for a crowd or just two meals for two people.

You need one or two cans of Italian (seasoned with oregano, garlic and basil) tomatoes diced and pureed in blender or Ninja or food processor. (I have used Paul Newman's sauce).

One or two 8 oz. yogurt or Ricotta cheese (preferred)

One egg or two eggs or Egg Beater if you use two Ricotta packages

Parsley - 2 tsp.

Cilantro fresh leaves cut off with scissors; two or three tbs.

Crushed garlic 1 tsp

Mix 8 oz. of yogurt or Ricotta with the egg and seasonings

Prepare your vegetables

2 small sliced zucchini, ½ shredded red cabbage,

1 or 2 packages thawed and drained frozen spinach.

Mushrooms - ½ cup

Kale leaves cut off the stem - ¼ cup

Vegetables can be varied but be sure to use mostly greens. Even if you do not like spinach, the sauce and cheese combinations and spices flavor will prevail.

Parmesan cheese grated to shake between layers of noodles.

8 oz. package of shredded mozzarella cheese.

Cook the desired amount of lasagna noodles while preparing the vegetables.

Heat oven to 350 degrees while layering your ingredients.

Use a glass square baking dish and assemble beginning with ½ cup of sauce in the bottom place a layer of noodles.

Spread ricotta mixture on top and add a thin spinach layer then alternate sauce, noodles, vegetables and cheeses.

Reserve a ½ cup of mozzarella for the top layer to be added the last 5 minutes of baking to melt the cheese. Bake uncovered for an hour.

Let stand for 15 minutes before cutting in squares to serve.

*TIP- make your sauce thick so the Lasagna does not run all over the plate. Remember the vegetables have water content. You can have some sauce on the side. Leftovers can be frozen in serving sizes for another delicious meal. You can add ground beef, sausage or turkey if you are feeding meat lovers. This recipe is very forgiving for a crowd or just two.

Spinach Omelet

I package thawed and drained spinach

4 small mini peppers chopped

1/4 red onion

½ c of mushroom pieces

2 eggs per person or ½ c of egg beaters

Sauté in olive oil or coconut oil, cut up peppers, red onion and mushrooms. Add the drained spinach. Pour your scrambled egg mixture in an omelet sized pan. Cook as you push cooked egg to the middle and let liquid egg flow to edges of the pan. When nearly done, add sautéed vegetables, drained spinach and fold over. When done add cheddar cheese to top and broil till melted. Serve with Salsa if desired.

Penne with a white sauce

You need for the sauce:

2 tbs of melted butter

Add 2 tbs. ground garlic

1 tbs. of flour to thicken

Add 3/4 cup chicken broth and 3/4 cup of milk

Cook on medium heat until desired thickness

Add 2 tsp of parsley flakes and 1/3 cup of Parmesan cheese

Salt and pepper to taste.

1 tbs. Cilantro on top when you serve.

Salad for Two

2 tomatoes, diced

4 medium carrots, sliced

2 celery stalks, sliced

½ small red onion, diced

6 sprigs of Cilantro leaves (fresh)

¼ cup of black olives

Add a dressing of olive oil and balsamic vinegar or lemon juice.

Nice when served in pita pockets (Syrian Bread)

*Tip- not too heavy on the dressing or your pockets will fall apart at the bottom. Warm in microwave for 30 Seconds so they separate easily. Stuff and enjoy!

Fruit dinner salad for two

½ head of lettuce

Apples ½ cup

Raspberries ½ cup (may use frozen)

Blueberries ½ cup

Dressing

½ cup plain yogurt

½ cup of Ricotta cheese

Mix with 1 tsp coconut oil

1 tbsp. lemon juice and 1 tbsp. of water

Pour over the salad.

Meat Pie

When I make stuffing I put aside some of the stuffing for a meat pie. I use ground turkey and ground sausage meat in my stuffing. Heat oven to 350 degrees.

Sauté in coconut oil ½ red onion 1 tsp. garlic.

When onion is transparent, remove from heat and snip the leaves from a kale stock and discard the stem. Mix with the onion and garlic. Add this to the Stuffing mix

Add ground cloves to taste. Approximately ⅛ tsp. Place mixture in a thawed pie shell.

Line the uncooked pie shell with 2 peeled, cored and sliced apples and place stuffing mix on the top. Bake at 350 for 35 minutes with tin foil covering the pie to prevent drying out and burning your crust. Remove foil to brown the crust the last ten minutes of baking time.

Serve on Christmas, Eve New Years with cranberry sauce, pickles, olives and celery. Or you can top it with cranberry trail mix. Some guest like it with just turkey gravy.

Brunch Quiche

Heat oven to 375.

Sauté in olive oil bell peppers, onions, and mushroom. Add garlic to taste and 2 handfuls of fresh spinach. Approximately ½ cup or more. Cover until vegetables are soft 3-5 minute. Let cool some.

Mix together the following in a bowl:

1 cup ricotta cheese

1 cup of Greek cheese or drained Yogurt

4 eggs, well beaten may substitute Egg Beaters

1 tsp nutmeg

3 tsp ground sage

Add the cooked vegetables and fold in with egg mixture.

Pour into uncooked pie shell and cover with tin foil loosely to prevent burning crust and drying out

Bake 40 45 minutes.

This recipe is compliments of Brain Research Labs.

Veggie side dish

Heat your frying pan and sauté small chopped bell peppers, red, yellow, and orange, ½ lb. green string beans and ½ red onion in Olive oil.

Add 1 cup of diced tomatoes with garlic, basil, and oregano (I use Great Value Italian diced tomatoes) to partially cooked peppers, add mushrooms and sliced zucchini if you like. Place green beans on the top with enough liquid to steam the beans when covered. Add snipped kale leaves on the top. You can use chicken broth for the liquid.

Side dishes

Cooked beet greens served with vinegar and oil.

Sliced cooked cold beats served pickled.

Cucumber slices and shoestring sliced carrots in vinegar and oil.

Healthy pancakes

Heat your fry pan with one tbsp. of coconut oil while mixing equal amounts of Bisquick, ground oatmeal (use a coffee grinder) and ground barley. If you add ground flax seed it makes the pancakes swell and will require more milk after sitting. Add 1 egg and use a whisk to mix well. Egg substitute works as well.

For variations, add sliced bananas after cooking, vary the syrup with frozen blueberries, and frozen strawberries. You can use cranberry trail mix with nuts as well.

Place syrup in the microwave for 30 seconds, longer if you use frozen fruit.

For lighter pancakes add ½ tsp baking powder. For richer pancakes add 1 tbsp. of coconut oil.

TIPS:

I am not a lover of duck, goose, anchovies, sardines, or oysters, but they are recommended by The Memory Healer Program (available on the internet to download).

I do like to make shrimp scampi in those little microwave dishes with the covers and vents sold in the dollar store now and then. They were advertising them on TV for $10.00 each.

Shellfish is not allowed for those trying to reduce cholesterol.

If dieting, eat the lowest Glycemic Index fruits that are loaded with vitamin C (for the brain): cherries, strawberries, tangerines, and oranges.

The goal is to add as much variety of fruits and vegetables. Have small servings of meats. Eliminate as many canned food and junk foods as possible. After 21 days the cravings for junk foods will be gone. You have unlimited choices from the fresh vegetable and fruit aisle. Fresh fish is a plus.

Most frozen fish today is packed in China. They do not have as strict laws on food packers as we do in this country. I have noticed some canned foods are packed in foreign countries too.

Caring for an Alzheimer's patient is time consuming. One of my time savers is to sit down with a cookbook and a cup of tea when he is napping. I make out a weekly menu and figure out what I can substitute to make the recipe brain healthy. From my weekly menu I do my grocery list. I shop early in the morning when there is fewer customers. Early in the week is when you will find things on sale.

Smoothies:

One of my favorite smoothies is made in a food processor from watermelon, ½ grapefruit and a few strawberries. Blend to a mush and eat with a spoon or add apple juice for a drink.

Another variation is adding blueberries instead of the grapefruit or add apple Juice for a refreshing drink with mint.

Green Smoothie by Vida Lexus

Start with spinach and kale in your blender. Add blueberries and strawberries and a banana for sweetness one half apple, one half pear, 2 tbsp. Bee Pollen 2 tbsp. ground Flaxseed and Almond Milk for liquefying to the liquid consistency desired or eat with a spoon.

There is no limit on what you can have as long as you are heavy on greens cooked on low heat steamed or raw to retain the most benefit.

Plenty of dairy including real butter, yogurt, cheeses and fruit. Sorry, but dairy is not good if you are trying to lower cholesterol. One percent milk has only 10 mg. of Cholesterol. Evaporated milk has no cholesterol and can be substituted in chowders, puddings and coffee instead of milk. The low cholesterol cheeses are cottage and mozzarella.

There has been some research done suggesting that keeping cholesterol in check is brain healthy so read your labels and decide what brands suit the needs of your loved one. I have found Skippy peanut butter is all natural without hydrogenated oil, preservatives or artificial coloring.

I buy additional fresh vegetables and fruit and process some whenever I have the time and extra produce. My pressure cooker only holds 4 pints at a time but it only takes about ten minutes to preserve food for enjoying when they are out of season.

Chapter 13
The Amish Have the Secret

We cannot all hold our jobs and continue our lifestyle and take care of an Alzheimer's patient. The Amish way of life may be too severe for most of us. We don't have to grow our own vegetables and raise our own meat to stay healthy the way the Amish do. We can tweak our way of living. Yes, making adjustments for the unwanted Alzheimer's disease takes effort, but the improvement you will see after time is well worth it. We all have access to organically grown produce. The internet offers more information than we can absorb. Just getting back to basics is a huge benefit.

I am not claiming a cure, only making life a bit easier to deal with - and in the process, buying some time to avoid confinement. Who knows, with all the research that is being done, Alzheimer's disease may be a manageable disease as well as other neurological ailments in the near future. If you think it is rough for you to deal with, have compassion for the patient coping with it. It has to be frightening to not know where you are or trying to make your needs known and you can't express yourself clearly. Not recognizing your loved ones or not remembering their names has to be frustrating. I truly hope my experience will be a help and I pray fervently that we see a breakthrough for Alzheimer's disease before the next generation is affected. If one lives long enough, there is an old person in their future.

I continue to do research and keep up with the latest herbal products and drugs. It is imperative that you only introduce one thing for 30 days or more before adding something else to give you an opportunity to see the results. If your patient is on multiple medications the doctor may have to adjust dosages of the medications until they are replaced with herbal products. It is of utmost importance to have a physician that is willing to work with you - if not, there are holistic doctors.

I have recently found Curcu Active powder that has scientifically shown to repair damaged synapses. The synapse is the electrical impulse that transmits thought from one neuron to the other. Without healthy synapse function, all the other supplements have limited benefits. There has been a slight recent memory improvement, but it is less than a month of taking this. There are many other health benefits from this powder that you add to your morning coffee. It is tasteless and odorless.

Everything that I am giving him is easy to find, order and research on the internet. You may find some in your health food store, but I didn't get out of the house too often, so I ordered online. Now that he has improved, I am able to get to my neighborhood health food store. They tend to offer some vegetables that are just not available in the big chain stores. I love the huge Portobello mushrooms

His lab work other, than his cholesterol, was normal. We have replaced eggs with Egg Maker or Egg Beater and do not consume red meat. Anything that is labeled greater than 10 mg. of cholesterol per serving we replace or omit. We only have shellfish once a year when we are treated with lobster on New Year's Day.

I am not married to a stranger anymore. He is not 100% of his former self, but he's made a huge improvement over the stranger of four years ago. I am grateful for that. My goal is to keep him home and functioning as long as possible. In the meantime, I pray for total reversal.

Chapter 14
Herbal Products Update for A.D.

1. Curcu Active powder to rebuild synapses to improve memory. Dissolve in coffee or juice. It is tasteless and dissolves well.
2. Neurocholine for cognition
3. Lion's Mane for memory
4. Bacopa relaxation and memory.
5. Procera A.V.H. behavior
6. Phosphatidyl Serine improves mental function

A total of six herbs are used to repair or replace damaged brain cells; combined with the right diet and purified water, we are seeing improvement.

Vitamins B6 normalizes homocysteine levels to prevent heart attacks by 73% (Miracles from the Vault) - it is also preventative for Alzheimer's disease.

B12 for memory, Folic Acid for mental clarity.

Recent studies have shown high incidence of mental symptoms associated with Folate deficiencies in the aged such as depression and dementia - including Alzheimer's disease.

It is painful to watch a productive, talented, thoughtful and fun-loving family member deteriorate to child-like behavior and ability.

To prevent Alzheimer's disease one could safely conclude, as evidenced by the research of experts, that taking Vitamin B supplements daily is a preventative step in the right direction.

Cod Liver oil with vitamin A and D - one a day has multiple benefits, especially for cardiac and brain health. It is an excellent source for Omega three.

Organic fruit and vegetable smoothies between meals are a boost to health and maintain healthy weight.

He also takes Turmeric Supreme for Arthritis. I have increased the dose to three a day when he has increased pain associated with weather changes. This has pepper extract to insure absorption at the cell level where it is needed. For inflammation, as stated in a previous chapter, Turmeric is being researched for other conditions as well, including brain health.

D3 10,000IU for psoriasis and brain function.

Citicoline (trade name Cognizen) for increased mental energy and neuroprotective benefits of brain cells.

I use the purified water in anything that will be eaten with the water in it to control the ingestion of fluorides and metals. Examples: rice and oatmeal (where water is absorbed).

I do not believe in statin drugs. A documented side effect is muscular weakness - and the heart is a muscle. It is safer to adjust the diet and remove red meat, eggs and shellfish.

My advice is to keep a log of what you are doing and the effect it has on the patient.

Do not discontinue any of their medications without approval of the doctor who ordered it. If your loved one is on several medications, be sure to include the list of herbal preparations.

You need to be active in their medication schedule as your loved one is not able. It is important to pay close attention to little changes. Keep literature on everything in a folder and include dates in your log. Document! Document! Document! There can be no disputing success or results when you have good records.

Part III
The Caretaker

Chapter 15
Caregiver's Concerns

When purchasing herbal products be sure to read the ingredients. If you buy from a different source you may find it under a different brand, but you will be getting the same thing or close to it.

A family member needs to address legal matters such as living wills and power of attorney. Those decisions should be made with the patient as early as possible.

Does the patient have advance directives? It puts a burden on other family members to make all the decisions regarding legal, health and financial issues.

It is important to have power of attorney from the patient prior to the disease advancing to a point that they are unable to make rational decisions.

Many decisions will have to be made in the future regarding the wishes of the patient including end of life decisions. Being prepared averts you having to make choices while grieving. It is best to have the patient's wishes in writing, preferably by their attorney.

As a caretaker it is important to take care of yourself. We have to decide when to arrange for respite care when we need help. We all get "burned out" at times because we are the chief cook, bottle washer, as well as functioning in the servant and nurse role. This can be pretty exhausting. Even an afternoon off to do an activity for your own pleasure will be a welcome reprieve.

I text or call each of my six children once or twice a week. This prevents feelings of isolation. I also keep up with what is going on with Facebook.

Schedule your life like you would for a new baby. In other words, do what you need to do when they sleep. Take a nap yourself in the afternoon or just have a quiet time with a cup of tea.

I have made the budget adjustments, such as cutting our own hair, coloring mine, doing my own nails. This is not much of a sacrifice because our social life is limited to going to church and the grocery store, and occasional visits with our daughter who lives close by.

I dread the day we have to clean the attic. He saves everything, including the broken items that he was able to fix in the past. Some repairs on the house will have to wait.

I have not yet contacted any support group. I looked into Alzheimer's facilities and found them to be very costly - even with veterans' benefits. Unless you have insurance for long term care, be prepared to pay two thousand dollars a month on the low side and significantly more in some areas. It is my hope that this will not be necessary.

At some point I will have to put the house up for sale, as well as a second automobile that has been collecting dust in the garage. It seems that we spend a lifetime collecting things and then we have the task of getting rid of our possessions. If we don't, our children will be burdened with this unnecessary obligation.

There are programs available through organizations to lighten the load. Every area is different, so look into what is available early on.

My children are a blessing to me for all their help and encouragement. This book evolved from keeping record for their future should they need it. Somewhere along the way I was encouraged by them to write a book.

Chapter 16
A Caregiver's Prayer

Heavenly Father, help me better understand and believe I can do what you ask me to do. Forgive me for the times, even now, when I question your judgment. As I go about the many daily tasks of caregiving, give me energy.

As I watch my loved one oh-so-slowly walk across the room, give me strength. As I answer his/her repeated question just one more time, give me patience. As I look for solutions to whatever is the most recent concern, give me wisdom. As I reminisce with him/her about the "good old days," give me a moment of laughter. As I get to know my loved one in a new way, seeing both his/her strength and frailty, give me joy. As I sit beside my loved one's bed waiting for his/her pain medication to take effect, give me comfort. Lighten my burden, answer my prayer, and give me the strength to do what so often seems impossible. Give me a quiet place to rest when I need it and a quieting of my anxieties when I'm there. Change my attitude from a tired, frustrated and angry caregiver to the loving and compassionate one I want to be. Remain my constant companion as I face the challenges of caregiving and when my job is through and it's time for me to let go, help me remember he/she is leaving my loving arms to enter your eternal embrace.

Amen

Borrowed from - www.youragingparent.com

About the Author
Phyllis Lozeau

Phyllis is a retired Registered Nurse. Her nursing career began in Obstetrics and ended as a charge nurse in a rehabilitation hospital. She is experienced in medical and surgical from pediatrics to elderly care nursing. Phyllis has been married for sixty years. She and Robert have six adult children, nine grandchildren and seven great grandchildren. She graduated from St. Joseph's School of Nursing and earned her Bachelor of Science Degree from Rivier College in New Hampshire. She diligently studied and pursued getting her degree while working in her husband's business in home building and pool construction.

While settling in Florida, she decided to learn technology, as well as the advances medicine had made in her absence. Now she is putting that knowledge to work as she focuses on caring for her husband during his battle with Alzheimer's disease.

Phyllis hopes that by sharing Robert's story and the treatments that are helping him improve and enhance his quality of life, that others suffering from the same condition can find comfort and improvement themselves.

www.ingramcontent.com/pod-product-compliance
Lightning Source LLC
Chambersburg PA
CBHW071221280526
45787CB00002B/749